WILL BOZEMAN

MILLION DOLLAR NURSES

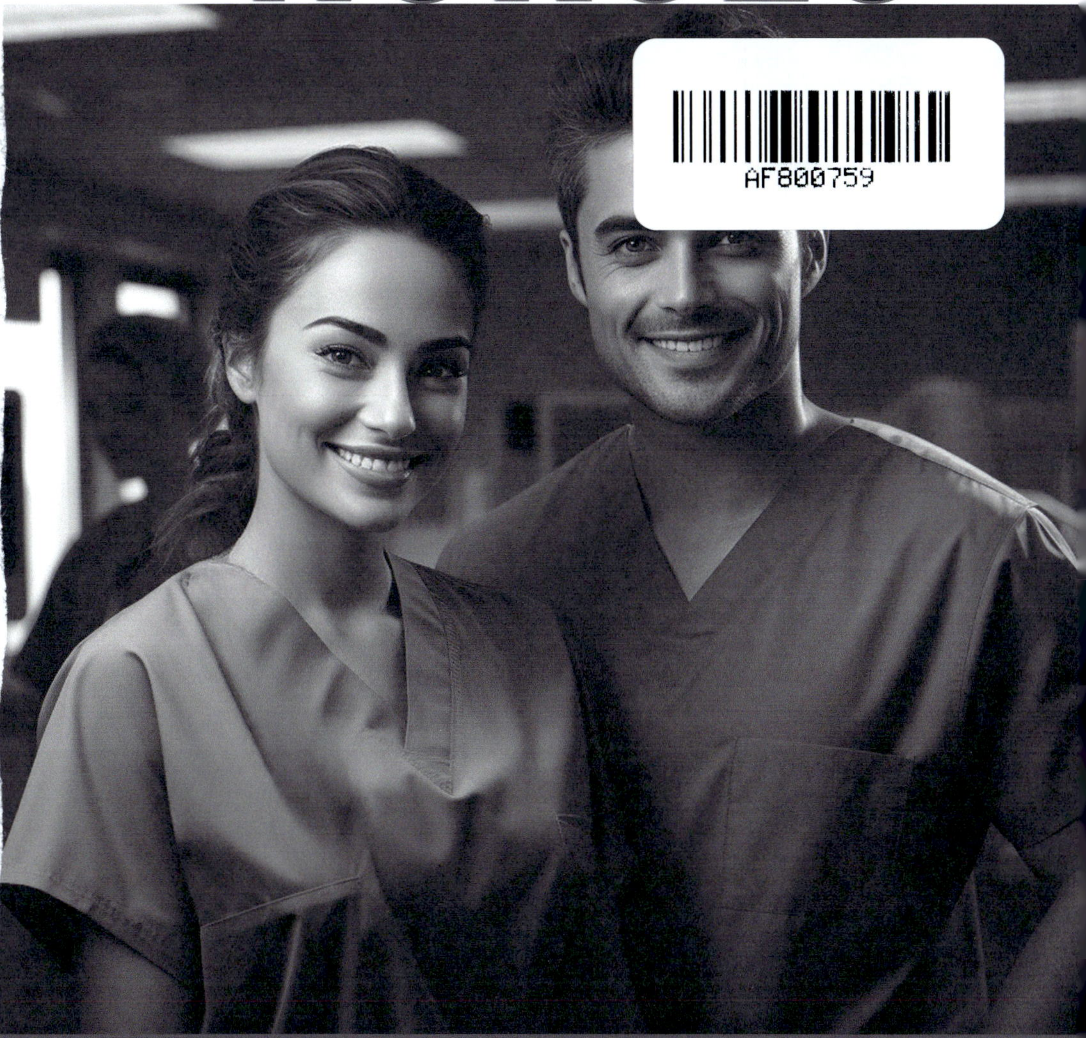

Launch your own mobile pain treatment business and love your job again!

Million Dollar Nurses

ISBN: 978-1-963592-24-5
ISBN: 978-1-963592-25-2
ISBN: 978-1-963592-26-9

Published by RELATYV Media

For more information:
http://www.willbozeman.com

Table of Contents

Gale's Story

Gale hobbled in on her four-post walker, with someone helping her as well, through the door of our new pain treatment practice that offered non-pharmaceutical, non-surgical, non-invasive pain treatment. Her neurologist had never heard of us or what we offered for treatment, but because it sounded safe enough, he approved her to get treatment. Gale had crippling peripheral neuropathy for over 25 years, and she had tried everything. She'd been working with this particular neurologist for most of that time. He agreed to let her get treatment with us because he couldn't increase her medications, she was ineligible for any other interventions like implants and surgeries, and so he approved her to move forward almost as a kind gesture to her, to let her feel like she was doing something for herself because he was out of options. He obviously believed nothing would come from this. In his mind, if there were a treatment that would work, he would have known about it and he would have offered it already, as per the mental plight of many experts, but that's another story. So, Gale is moving forward with our treatment program as a last-ditch effort for something to work.

Halfway through the program she started coming to the office without her four-post walker and only using a single post cane. This alone was a tremendous success for her! Everyone was impressed and she couldn't believe it! She didn't stop there, she kept going. Weeks of treatment went by and on the last day of treatment she walked into the office with no walker, lightly stepped to the middle of the room in front of all the other patients who were in pain and danced a little jig of success for everyone to see. She said, "This is what you have to look forward to!" She inspired all those patients to keep going in the program. Really though, she inspired us because we'd never seen transformations like this and the nurses and staff in the office didn't know what to think!

A few months later Gale walks into the office, no walkers, and everyone is really happy to see her and she's smiling and talking with everyone. She opened her wallet and pulled out her brand-new driver's license! She hadn't been able to drive in over 20 years and she had just requalified to start driving again after getting out of pain and being able to feel her legs and feet again! Her whole life changed. Her entire trajectory of health went from downward to upward, from negativism to optimism, and from despair to hope!

What's this life changing treatment I'm talking about? Neurofunctional Pain Management. A safe and simple combination treatment protocol I developed using known and proven technology and known and proven techniques restructured into a combination therapy that were never fully applied and utilized in the world of pain management, or in medicine at all. Sometimes it takes an outsider to see what's on the inside, and in this case, I was in the right place at the right time to see something that was right in front of everyone, yet nobody knew what they had.

Since then, I created a mission statement that I feel really captures the essence of the program for Neurofunctional Pain Management: Relieve Pain, Restore Health, and Magnify Quality of Life.

In this book I'm going to show you the tremendous opportunity available in the world of mobile pain care using Neurofunctional Pain Management that will create a whole new career field for nurses and other credential medical care professionals.

I'm going to show you how strong the need is for this treatment and how tens of millions of patients are not ambulatory enough to get into offices and access treatment, opening the door for mobile pain treatment.

I'll show you how to use your current credentials and structure yourself as the mobile technician who can step in and offer this service and get paid nicely for it.

I'll also show you how you can build your own business operation to earn over a million dollars a year, making you a Million Dollar Nurse!

Ready? Let's dive in!

Personal Backstory from Gale

In 2008 I lost four jobs in a row! It was one of the hardest times in my life financially. I had just graduated from college, just gotten married, and had a job I didn't even like in a field I didn't even go to school for. Yes, I even got let go from that job within days after getting married! I've never been one to sit still for long, so I was back out looking for another job that very day. I found one! Then after three months they closed down and I was back on the hunt. I found another! Then they cut staff after three months and I was last man in, so first one out. I found another job in a completely different field and yes, it only lasted three months before they cut back as well.

I was at the mercy of everyone else and I hated feeling that way! I could get another job, and then I'd be entirely dependent on them to "take care of me" as long as I was valuable to them. I decided right then that I'd never let my future depend on someone else.

"The main difference between working for yourself and working for someone else is that if you work for yourself, you know how long you have left." Will Bozeman

I started telling people this after I realized that I didn't know how long I had left in any of these other jobs I lost, but the owners and managers did. They can see the financial writing on the wall weeks and months before they actually let someone go. I hated the idea of not knowing if I was a "dead man walking" at work and still trying to spin my wheels for someone else all while they are calculating how long they have until they have to let me go. So, in my mind, when you own the company, you know how long you have. When you are an employee, you don't know until they tell you you're done.

After all those jobs and all that stress I launched my own Amazon store selling health supplements. I found a local manufacturer that was willing to let me buy their off-brand house label products, that were left over from large production runs for big brands and sell them on Amazon. I remember being so excited about that! I opened the Amazon seller account and started fumbling through the listing creation process. I finally got the listings up for the products I was carrying. I put everything up and then waited...and waited...and waited, and nothing. Days went by and I was a little bummed. I knew I wouldn't be a millionaire from selling these supplements, I just wanted a little money to pay the bills.

Finally, one day I was at a big family event with everyone around. I opened my email and there it was, Sold, Ship Now. I still get a little spark of dopamine when I see those words. Anyone out there who's ever had an Amazon seller account can attest to this! I'm sure some people reading this are enjoying their dopamine right now after seeing those words. So, naturally I set up my smart phone to ding with a cash register sound whenever I received a Sold, Ship Now email from my seller account. It was sooooo fun to be out and about and hear the "cha-ching" sound. Driving around town running errands, "cha-ching"! Playing games with friend and "cha-ching" and of course I'm so excited I can't wait for someone to ask me why I set my ring tone to that sound, but it didn't do that when I got a text? Hahaha, then I got to explain that I made a sale.

Back to the first sale, I stared at that order. It validated all that work and belief I had about this working. I structured all my products, so I'd have a pure $10 profit margin after all costs and fees, with every unit sold, so that email represented $10 in my pocket. I felt in that moment that

I could do great things, and I can accomplish what I want to accomplish in life. It's a feeling I wanted everyone else to feel and the more I am around people who hate their jobs the more I want to show them what's possible!

Fast forward a few months and I'm getting about 6-8 orders a day, sometimes single items, sometimes multiple items. One year later I'm getting about 40-50 orders a day. I remember being excited to do the packaging and shipping each night for the day's orders. People laugh when they hear this story because I was working full time and going to school full time at this point. I couldn't get to the manufacturer to pick up my sold inventory for shipping until after hours. So, the owners would bag up all my orders and put them out behind the recycle dumpster in the parking lot. I would drive over after classes, pick up my products, and head home to print labels and ship them. It was a fun cycle of work, and I actually really enjoyed filling the orders and thinking about all these customers and recognizing the re-orders and being really excited to see the same names and addresses coming through. This was just so fun for me. My wife at the time would head on to bed and I would stay up packing orders and watching TV and doing homework. Yeah, busy time of life but I enjoyed that work because it was my work.

Then I moved all that work to Amazon fulfillment so it could be listed as a Prime eligible purchase, and my sales shot up. Pretty soon I was making tens of thousands of dollars a month on autopilot. I set my system to automatically order inventory when it dropped to a certain count, it shipped, and Amazon stocked it and sold it. Suddenly my bills are all paid and I'm making great money while I'm in Disneyland with the family on vacation or while I'm sleeping at night. I wake up and I made $1000 overnight. I ignore my account for a week on vacation and come back and I made $5000.

It's this kind of freedom that I'd never experienced before. It allowed me to pursue other passions and even go back to school to get into the field that I had a passion for, biotechnology, and that's how I ended up in the medical field and the ability to write this book!

Why am I telling you this story?

I'll be the first person to relate to you about the dissatisfaction of working for someone else and never really knowing if I was secure, or feeling like I'm building something for them that doesn't' belong to me and hating that feeling. I think part of the W2 employment myth is that of protection and security. Sure, W2 provides some state benefits if you lose your job, but just because you're a W2 employee does not mean your job is secure. In fact, in my experience, it's the W2's who are first to go because the contractors can be worked with and negotiated with for payment terms and changes in the agreements. W2, not so much. They get paid what they get paid whether they perform or not, and they know this, so there's no incentive to perform, just to get paid. Even most incentive programs and bonus programs are insulting and pandering to the employee and don't make them work harder, just makes them resentful that they are being taunted to work harder with some extra bonuses. I've seen this happen several times where management conjures this idea to get people to care and work harder and be productive. Most of the time it just comes across as a carrot on a string and people will just ignore it. Then managers switch to using a stick to get the same upgrade in output and production and that just makes people angry, resentful, and afraid. None of these emotional connections to their work make you care like owning your own business and knowing that you are building something that's yours!

W2 employees are all too often only concerned with getting their paychecks. They don't think like a business owner, they think like a child with a parent that provides everything. As long as they make Mom and Dad happy, I'll get a treat, so be on my best behavior. I suppose ignorance is bliss for some people, but again, you can still be fired at any time and then all that ignorance and bliss goes right out the window, and you start thinking about how you NEVER want to experience this again!

So, that's why I'm telling you this story. There's no feeling in the working world like the one of knowing you are secure and that you make your own income happen, and that you don't have to dance and sing for your supper. You do have to work, and work hard, and that's what we're going to talk about here. You ARE working for this, but you'll get what you want! Security, protection, and- income that is all controlled by you!

Chapter 1

Chronic Pain in the US Today

Healthcare is going more and more mobile! Since covid there has been a boom in mobile and online telemedicine activity worldwide. Some types of medicine are well-suited for this, and some aren't easily able to expand into the mobile/telemed medical model. This opens the doors of opportunity for the right person in the right category of medicine to step through!

Pain management is one of these categories that has tremendous opportunity, need, and demand to expand into the mobile setting. Most pain doctors are moving toward procedures offered in facilities and surgery centers, as a primary objective. I know this because I've talked to hundreds of pain doctors over the years and with the growing public outcry over opioids, and the increased scrutiny of medication prescriptions, pain doctors are more and more likely to reduce prescriptions and move toward interventional modalities like procedures, blocks and injections, implants, and surgeries. None of which can be performed in a mobile setting.

In addition to this shift to interventional procedures, many of the patients who need these treatments can't easily get into the office for them, even with help and support. In my estimation roughly 25-50% of chronic pain patients out there are non-ambulatory. I created a LinkedIn poll to ask my physician community this very question: What percent of you pain patients are not ambulatory enough to get into the office for procedures? The answers are right where I knew they'd be. The vast majority of doctors who responded said 25-50% of their patients meet this description of being non-ambulatory and can't take advantage of the range of interventional procedures pain doctors are offering.

In comes the opportunity for a mobile service, but what actual service could be performed in a mobile setting that would actually help a pain patient like this? Neurofunctional Pain Management!

"According to the Centers for Disease Control and Prevention (CDC), 51.6 million US adults, or almost 21% of the population, experienced chronic pain in 2021. This is an increase from 20.5% to 21.8% between 2019 and 2021. Of those, 17.1 million adults, or 6.9%, experienced high-impact chronic pain, which can significantly limit their ability to work or participate in daily activities.

Chronic pain can affect quality of life and is a significant public health problem. It can cost society at least $560–635 billion annually, which is about $2,000 for every person in the US." Google AI Response

Full disclosure this is a simple google search with an automated AI explanation of the current data on pain management. It sounded good so I went ahead and added it here.

OK, so let's do a little math here. 21% of the population is over 51 million people. Let's assume half are not dealing with debilitating chronic pain, but are managing it on their own, that's 25 million people. Let's now use that stat from pain offices that roughly half their patients aren't ambulatory enough to get into the office and that leaves us with 12.5 million patients in chronic pain who would benefit and likely need/want a mobile treatment option for their chronic pain.

You can keep doing the math here, but that basically means over 5% of the people in your town or city are dealing with this very problem. You live in a town of 10,000 people? That's 500 people in that situation.

You'll learn later in the book that a full load of patients for a mobile pain treatment nurse engaged in Neurofunctional Pain Management is only about 15 at any given time, so in a town of 10,000 people there's easily a need for a dozen nurses engaged in this program, of course assuming that all these patients are in treatment, but even just a modest acceptance of this program by the medical community in a town of 10,000 people there would be a need for several nurses. This is an excellent situation for you because I'll show you how this is an advantage for you in growing your business to serve that need!

I probably don't need to keep explaining the need here. Everyone knows chronic pain is an epidemic crisis level category and as you can see above, it costs the US economy hundreds of billions a year annually in direct cost to treat and in lost productivity in the labor field so, there is absolutely a need for this and you can fill that demand and build a successful business that can change your life and help you love what you do again!

Chapter 2

A pain treatment program that works

OK, so I'm not a nurse. I went to medical school in Alabama for two years and I took a leave of absence to join a biotech startup in Arizona as their Chief Science Officer. The story about the Amazon store above factors into this path. I went back to school and got a second undergrad in Biotechnology. I also completed all the requirements to go to medical school, took the MCAT and did decent enough to land a spot in medical school. I carried my Amazon store the whole time and it paid for all this because I owned my own business.

I took a leave of absence from medical school to open that biotech venture, and I had way too much fun building that company, and I decided not to go back and finish med school. I've been in the biotech and medical business field ever since. Luckily, my biotech company worked with pain management, so I was lecturing and presenting at conferences for those years that I was the science officer. It was great and I learned a lot about the field of pain management.

I stumbled across an interesting electrical device. It produced a high pulse electrical current that depolarized pain neurons and produced a pain relief effect. Did I mention my first degree path in college was electrical engineering? My associates degree before my first undergrad was in electrical engineering and I worked as an electrician for a couple years, off and on, during my college years, that and I delivered pizza in the evenings for years in college as well, so I do have a little experience in the whole mobile business concept! Back to the story, I love electricity and electrical concepts, and I love biotechnology and medicine, so I was totally hooked on the concept of electrical therapies and neuromodulation.

The first thing I learned was that not all these devices are the same! You should understand that right now. MOST doctors can't describe the difference between one pulsation therapy and another, nor can they describe or care to understand the details of how those different currents impact cells and tissues. They just do what the manual says and what the rep for the device tells them. There's a tremendous amount of difference between devices.

Electroanalgesia vs Transcutaneous Electrical Nerve Stimulation (TENS) – I've written several articles about this very topic because it's extremely common for doctors to be confused about the differences and why one will work and the other won't for various intended outcomes. If the doctors are confused, then I guarantee the patients have no clue what's going with it. TENS units have a pulse per second range between 1-450pps. The FDA classifies devices by their pulse per second capacity and that determines where they fall in the world of medical devices. TENS units are low power devices that make them safe to use in non-medical offices like PT and Chiropractic offices, you can even buy lower power versions for home use inexpensively on Amazon. Electroanalgesia devices are able to achieve many thousands of pulses per second, much more powerful than a TENS unit, and much more therapeutically beneficial for a wide range of things. The devices we use in Neurofunctional Pain Management go up to 10,000pps and can directly impact pain neurons at that level.

Now that you know that difference, why don't you see more doctors using these devices? Well, reason number one, it takes a lot of time and effort to do a treatment program using this therapy. You need to engage a patient in a treatment program at least twice a week for several weeks to obtain an enduring effect. I experimented with this variety of possible treatment cycles and landed on the following that seems to work really well. Two 1hr treatment events per week for 8 weeks. What would a patient expect from this?

Our doctors have reported that 85% of the patients we treat in the program have achieved a greater than 50% reduction in pain. Keep in mind that these are chronic pain patients that likely have been in pain for years and decades. Getting a 10-20% reduction would be considered a win by most doctors, so for us to get that much of a result is amazing. To top that off, about 30-40% of patients will achieve a fully resolved or nearly resolved pain outcome, meaning that they are either pain free or nearly pain free at the end of the program. This is also incredibly valuable to the medical community!

Here's the next aspect of incredible info about these results. Patients who complete the program will likely see an enduring result of pain relief of 3-6 months after completing the program. This means that they don't need any additional treatment or interventional therapies to achieve several months of ongoing relief. It's not uncommon for patients to go 6-12 months pain free after treatment and I have had patients come back into my offices over a year after completing treatment to tell us they are still out of pain! I've never heard of anything else in pain management that can produce a year long result without any additional intervention or interaction, no pills, no injections, no nothing and the pain relief endures for a year?!?

"Why in the world have I nor heard of this?"

With results like this I have heard this question from literally hundreds of patients and dozens of doctors and staff. Why haven't I ever heard of this or seen this before?

Workload, time, and reimbursement. If you're a busy pain doctor you don't have time to do what I just described above. Spend 16 hours over

8 weeks with one patient treating them in this program. You also don't want to pay your staff to do this, and almost more importantly, you don't have space in your office for this, and for these many patients cycling through your office 16 times over 8 weeks. So...this is likely why you don't see it much. In fact, I know doctors who have the devices in their offices and only use it as a back up in case the other options don't work!!!

So, let' me just restate that for you so you hear me very clearly. Many of the pain doctors I know who have an electroanalgesia treatment device in their office will wait until the steroid injections and pain pill stop working before, they will consider getting the patient on a course of electroanalgesia treatment!!! So, they are literally saving the conservative therapy option until last, because they know it will work so they save it for last in case the other stuff doesn't work. I kid you not I have been baffled by hearing this from some doctors I've talked to.

Also, another reason for not doing it, consider the reimbursement on this. Doctor spends an hour and makes $150 on this treatment. Doctor spends 15min on a spinal injection and makes $600. So, four spinal injections an hour equals $2400 an hour for treatments. That's 16 times more money per hour than doing this treatment. So, now let's ask that question again, why have I not seen this before? That's why, because doctors can make tremendously more, 16 times more, for the time spent by not doing this treatment. So, they don't do it, they don't offer it, and they don't even recommend or suggest it unless everything else fails to work for the patient because it's just not worth their time to engage in it.

BUT it is definitely worth YOUR time as a mobile pain treatment nurse, and I'll explain why this is the case below.

Fast-forward a few years and I found myself opening medical offices that I owned and hiring physicians to run them medically while I ran and oversaw them on the business side. Having a medical background really helped me interact with doctors, nurses, and staff. Most doctors even said I made the right move because they were generally unhappy with their situation in the medical field. I quickly found that most doctors weren't too happy about their situation. I kept digging into that concept that most doctors aren't happy in their current situation.

If doctors aren't happy, then who else is unhappy? Nurses and nearly all the other staff I encountered, that's who! I asked questions and I found a lot of answers. But before I jump into all that let's talk about the thing that tipped the delicate apple cart of medical office work a few years ago!

Chapter 3

Covid 19 and The Nurse Rush

I suppose I don't have to tell you anything about this! We all just lived through it, so we all know how everything changed, but let me tell you, my experience. In my state, all non-essential and elective medical treatment and procedures were halted. I owned and operated pain treatment centers so those actually qualified as essential because people are still in pain, so we stayed open.

We had a tremendous inflow of patients because there were only a few places open and seeing patients. The main problem we had was finding staff! Everyone was snapped up in the covid staff rush. We had ads going for months with no responses. We were looking for MA's and couldn't get anyone to apply. When we did get an application, we would do a phone call and you know what they would ask right at the beginning? "How much are you offering?" They knew what was going on and they knew they were valuable.

This story of my experience was mostly regarding MA's, but it was the same story with nurses and pretty much all medical professional staff. MA's pay easily doubled within a few months. I asked some of them what it would take to get them to come on board and I would hear things like $30/hr, $35/hr, and I believe we had one MA that said she'd only switch over to us for $40, but I was not on that call and my partner, who was a seasoned doctor with 20 years of experience in running offices, just laughed about that all day. The going rate for an entry level MA in my area in 2019 was $15-17/hr. So having to compete at $30-40 was really hard to manage, especially when the work we were doing wasn't paying more than it was a year ago, in fact like most years the reimbursement rates for our work had ticked down a little, as per the norm, but the labor pricing spiked in a very short time.

So where does that leave us now?

> "Travel nurses took high-paying jobs during Covid. But then their pay was slashed, sometimes in half."
>
> NBC News

This news article headline kinda sums up the employment scenario that covid caused. All those pay rates I just mentioned above didn't last, they can't last, because they are inconsistent with how much medical offices and primary care offices actually make and can afford to pay staff. Emergency funds allowed all these hospitals and groups to compete for limited available staff, so the pay rates when up, way up, then fell back down after the emergency aid was cut.

Of course, the pay increase was justified for covid, I'm not suggesting nurses should have been paid the same, I'm just trying to paint the landscape here and help people understand the changes. Here are the main reasons why pay needed to increase during the pandemic:

1. **Increased Workload and Stress**

   Overwhelming Patient Load: The pandemic led to a surge in patients, particularly in critical care settings, overwhelming healthcare systems and forcing nurses to manage a significantly higher number of patients, often under intense pressure.

   Emotional Toll: Nurses faced not only the physical demands but also the emotional strain of caring for severely ill and dying patients in unprecedented numbers, often without the comfort of family presence.

2. **Exposure to Health Risks**

   Increased Risk of Infection: Nurses were on the front lines, frequently exposed to the virus, which heightened their risk of contracting COVID-19. The initial shortage of personal protective equipment (PPE) exacerbated this risk, leading to widespread anxiety and fear among healthcare workers.

   Long-Term Health Effects: Some nurses who contracted COVID-19 suffered long-term effects, impacting their ability to work and their overall health.

3. **Shift in Job Roles and Responsibilities**

   Expanded Responsibilities: The pandemic required nurses to take on expanded roles, including conducting COVID-19 testing, administering vaccines, and managing patient care in rapidly changing and often chaotic environments.

   Cross-Training: Many nurses were cross-trained to work in different units or specialties to meet the demands of the crisis, sometimes moving from general wards to intensive care units with little preparation.

4. **Psychological Impact**

   Increased Burnout: The prolonged stress, coupled with the emotional toll of witnessing so much suffering and death, led to a significant increase in burnout, anxiety, and depression among nurses.

   Moral Distress: Nurses often faced moral dilemmas, such as rationing care or working in conditions where they felt patient safety was compromised, leading to moral distress and job dissatisfaction.

5. **Changes in Staffing and Workforce Dynamics**

   Staff Shortages: The pandemic exacerbated existing nursing shortages, with some nurses leaving the profession due to burnout, illness, or fear of exposure, leading to even greater staffing challenges.

   Increased Reliance on Travel Nurses: To cope with shortages, many healthcare facilities turned to travel nurses, leading to a more transient workforce and changes in team dynamics.

6. **Telehealth and Remote Work**

   Expansion of Telehealth: The pandemic accelerated the adoption of telehealth, with some nurses transitioning to remote roles, conducting patient assessments, and providing care via virtual platforms. This shift required nurses to adapt to new technologies and ways of interacting with patients.

   Remote Nursing Roles: Some administrative and case management roles shifted to remote work, offering nurses more flexibility but also requiring adjustments to communication and collaboration.

7. **Changes in Patient-Nurse Interaction**

   Limited Family Interaction: With strict visitation policies in place, nurses often became the primary point of contact between patients and their families, adding emotional responsibilities to their roles.

   Communication Challenges: Wearing PPE made communication with patients more difficult, leading to challenges in building rapport and providing comfort.

8. **Impact on Professional Development**

   Disruption of Education and Training: Many educational and professional development opportunities were postponed or moved online, impacting ongoing learning and career advancement for nurses.

Adaptation to Rapid Changes: Nurses had to quickly adapt to evolving guidelines, protocols, and treatments related to COVID-19, often with limited training or support.

9. **Work-Life Balance Challenges**

Increased Work Hours: Many nurses worked extended hours or multiple shifts due to staff shortages and increased patient load, leading to exhaustion and difficulties in maintaining a work-life balance.

Isolation and Quarantine: Some nurses faced periods of isolation or quarantine after exposure, leading to personal and professional disruptions.

COVID-19 has had a profound impact on the nursing profession, highlighting both the resilience and vulnerabilities of nurses in the healthcare system. One thing I will talk about later is the realization that there is a limitation for nurses on income and career advancement. Really, the only way to make more money, and it's not a whole lot more money, is to take on more responsibility with more stress.

Pay increases during covid versus now

I dug up a few stats and details on the pay changes for nurses during and after covid, so here are some details:

1. **Travel Nurses**

Substantial Pay Increases: Travel nurses, who were deployed to areas with critical shortages, saw some of the most significant pay increases. In some cases, their pay tripled compared to pre-pandemic levels. Reports indicated that travel nurses were earning upwards of $5,000 to $10,000 per week during the peak of the pandemic, especially in hotspots like New York City or California.

Signing and Completion Bonuses: Many travel nursing contracts included signing bonuses, completion bonuses, and other incentives to attract nurses to high-need areas.

2. **Hospital and Permanent Staff Nurses**

Temporary Pay Raises and Bonuses: Many hospitals offered temporary hazard pay, bonuses, and increased hourly wages to retain permanent staff nurses. Some nurses reported pay increases of 20-50% over their regular salaries during the height of the pandemic.

Overtime and Shift Differentials: With many nurses working extended hours and multiple shifts, overtime pay, and shift differentials (for night or weekend shifts) also contributed to increased earnings.

3. **Intensive Care Unit (ICU) and Specialized Nurses**

Higher Pay for Specialized Roles: ICU nurses and those with specialized skills, such as those working with ventilators or in COVID-19 units, often received higher pay due to the critical nature of their work. Their hourly wages increased significantly, with some hospitals offering double or triple the normal rates.

4. **Hazard Pay and Bonuses**

Hazard Pay: Some healthcare facilities introduced hazard pay as a temporary measure to compensate nurses and other frontline medical staff for the increased risk of working during the pandemic. This typically amounted to an additional $10 to $25 per hour, depending on the facility and region.

Retention Bonuses: To retain staff, especially in areas with severe shortages, hospitals and healthcare systems offered retention bonuses, which could range from several hundred to several thousand dollars.

5. **Regional Variations**

   Urban vs. Rural Differences: Pay increases were generally more pronounced in urban areas and COVID-19 hotspots compared to rural regions. Urban hospitals facing severe outbreaks had to offer competitive wages to attract and retain staff, whereas rural areas saw more modest increases.

   State-by-State Differences: States with higher COVID-19 case numbers or stricter regulations often saw more significant pay increases for nurses and medical staff.

6. **Temporary Contracts and Crisis Pay**

   Crisis Pay: Some nurses took on temporary or crisis contracts that offered significantly higher pay due to the urgent need for their skills. These contracts often came with higher base pay, bonuses, and additional benefits like housing stipends.

7. **Impact on Support Staff**

   Incremental Raises: While nurses saw the most significant pay increases, other medical staff, such as respiratory therapists, paramedics, and certified nursing assistants (CNAs), also experienced pay bumps, though typically not as dramatic. Support staff were often offered hazard pay and bonuses as well.

Post-Pandemic Adjustments

Decline in Crisis Pay: As the pandemic stabilized and the demand for crisis response diminished, many of these pay increases were scaled back. However, some permanent increases in base pay and benefits were implemented to reflect the ongoing need for a robust healthcare workforce.

There are a lot of details and scenarios, but ultimately the high pay that some nurses got used to during the pandemic no longer exists. Sure, there are some residual benefits of the pandemic still present in the regular work environment, but most of the high dollar benefits are gone and nurses are back to the grind with not a whole lot of hope for getting back to those high dollar incomes...until now, as I'll explain below.

Chapter 4

A Nurse in Today's Healthcare Environment

So, where are nurses and other nursing staff today regarding satisfaction? Yeah, my story about the doctors not being happy about their current employment scenario is the same for many nurses I talk to, and I've talked to a lot of nurses.

I have a whole list of reasons why, but I can tell you that there are options that can change how this works and how you can make excellent income and actually get a chance to connect with patients, changes lives, make a difference, and love what you do again!

Let's take a quick look at the top 10 list of reasons why nurses are unhappy in their current job. Keep in mind this isn't a top 10 list associated with covid, this is just regular nursing positions and regular work scenarios. Spoiler alert, I have a solution to all of these complaints that I'll outline below, but first I want to point them out for you, though I suspect you already know what they are, and you could write this list yourself:

1. **High Stress and Burnout**

   Nursing is inherently stressful, with long hours, high patient-to-nurse ratios, and the emotional toll of caring for sick or dying patients. This constant pressure can lead to burnout, affecting both mental and physical health.

2. **Inadequate Staffing**

   Chronic understaffing in many healthcare settings forces RNs to manage more patients than is safe or reasonable, increasing the risk of errors and reducing the quality of care, leading to frustration and job dissatisfaction.

3. **Lack of Autonomy**

   Many RNs feel they have little control over their work environment or decisions about patient care, often being required to follow strict protocols and orders from physicians or administrators, which can be demoralizing.

4. **Poor Work-Life Balance**

   Irregular hours, mandatory overtime, and rotating shifts are common in nursing, making it difficult to maintain a healthy work-life balance. This can strain personal relationships and lead to exhaustion.

5. **Limited Career Advancement**

   Career progression opportunities can be limited in traditional nursing roles, particularly for those who do not wish to move into management or administrative positions, leading to feelings of stagnation.

6. **Inadequate Compensation**

   Many RNs feel that their salaries do not adequately reflect the level of responsibility, expertise, and risk associated with their work. This feeling is exacerbated by the rising cost of living and student loan debt.

7. **Lack of Recognition and Appreciation**

   Nurses often feel undervalued and unappreciated by both patients and healthcare administrators. The lack of recognition for their hard work and dedication can be demoralizing.

8. **Physical Demands and Health Risks**

   The physical demands of nursing, including long hours on their feet, lifting patients, and exposure to infectious diseases, can lead to chronic health issues, pain, and injuries, contributing to job dissatisfaction.

9. **Administrative Burden**

   RNs are increasingly required to spend a significant amount of time on documentation and administrative tasks, reducing the time available for patient care. This shift in focus can be frustrating for those who entered the profession to care for patients.

10. **Moral Distress**

    RNs often face ethical dilemmas and situations where they feel unable to provide the level of care, they believe is necessary due to institutional constraints, leading to moral distress and job dissatisfaction.

OK, so you already know that these factors collectively contribute to a sense of frustration and unhappiness among RNs in traditional W-2 employment. I have solutions for all these problems in the program I'm about to explain.

Chapter 5

Benefits of a Mobile Pain Treatment Program

Remember that amazing pain treatment program I described earlier? Well, what if that program were converted into a mobile program that nurses could engage in? And on top of that, what if it paid really well, gave you autonomy in your work, allowed you to spend quality time with patients, allowed you to choose your own schedule, and even offered you continued opportunities to advance your work and business to grow into a substantially profitable operation that you own and operate yourself?

I'm chuckling as I write this because I know some of you are saying out loud right now, Yeah Right? I know you are because I know a lot of nurses and they have a highly refined bullshit-o-meter. So, I'll honor that meter and get straight to how this works.

This is a mobile pain treatment program that operates as an ancillary service to medical offices and doctors who have pain patients who are not ambulatory enough to make it into the office. Using Neurofunctional Pain Management like I described above, a patient can be treated for chronic pain in a home setting without having to go into the office. This means that there is a huge opportunity to step in and offer service for these doctors and offices. BUT, I'm not suggesting you step in and work as a W2 employee, I'm suggesting you structure yourself as an independent 1099 contractor who is paid for services performed. Effectively you are your own business, and you have sooo much more control over your work and life in this business model.

The underlying principle here is that there are chronic pain patients everywhere in the nation that desperately need this treatment and doctors can't get effective treatment for those patients. We're talking about a gap in the system with millions of patients and tens of thousands of nurses who could turn this into an opportunity to make a significant impact on helping these patients in chronic pain. Most of them are on medications or are being guided down a path to steroid injections, spinal cord implants, and surgeries of all kinds. You can be the shining light for these patients, offering them an option they likely were never presented or even heard about from their regular doctors and specialists.

Hey, all those pain medications, surgeries, and steroid injections exist for a reason and have a place in the medical cycle, but wouldn't it be best to try something that was conservative and highly effective first before doing all those other things and taking all those other risks? This is what I'm talking about here. Giving patients a way to success in pain relief without all the negative options out there in front of them.

I've asked a LOT of patients about what they would pick if they were presented with all these options, they hands down want to go with the least invasive and non-pharmaceutical option that will actually work. I say actually work because there are a lot of options out there that fall into the non-pharmaceutical and non-surgical category, but they are all very temporary and some of them are just wishful thinking efforts that require the patient to suffer as they keep trying to make it work. Neurofunctional Pain Management can actually have a significant success in pain relief after the first treatment, and of course, we're talking about a lasting effect that can last for months with no additional treatment, so this is a very significant and successful treatment protocol.

I want to explain a concept called HAVE TO GET TO. I know this concept existed before I lacked on to it, but the concept is exactly what it says. There's one feeling about something when you "have to" do it or engage in it, there's a different feeling about it when you "get to" do it or engage in it. Imagine going to Disneyland, assuming here that that's something fun you like and want to do. You "get to" go to Disneyland so you are excited, and you want to do it and can't wait! Now imagine that you "have to" go to Disneyland every day for the next year. At first it might feel like a "get to" scenario and you're excited about it, and you enjoy those first few days, but after riding all the same rides each day, seeing the same shows and parades each day, and eating the same food day after day? Six months into this that "get to" becomes a "have to", it becomes a chore. Now remember this as I'm going into the next section here.

OK, so I want to address each of these top 10 reasons for nurses being unhappy and show you how my program will overcome that issue:

1. **High Stress and Burnout**

    I think you can already imagine how what I'm proposing overcomes this issue but let me lay it out for you. As an independent contractor you choose your own work schedule. You don't have to do what you don't want to do. You're not "required" to work certain shifts or do certain types of work you don't like or make up the slack from other nurses. I put required in parenthesis because you still "have to" work, you just don't have people imposing their need on your like working a double shift or working nights or any other type of scenario like that. You are independent, so you set your schedule, and all this work converts to a "get to" situation and you're actually excited about it. You get excited to go to work.

    Literally, this will change your whole mindset of working. You control your work, and you will quickly become addicted to being able to manage your own schedule and drive your own ambition on this. I have another saying I love and live by, Entrepreneurs Love Mondays! You'll eventually feel the same way as you're making excellent money, and you have the ability to grow and build your new business into something more. Trust me, you'll start loving Mondays because everyone is back in action! Also, because you don't have to clock in at a job you can't stand. Just wait, you'll see it and feel it yourself!

2. **Inadequate Staffing**

I touched on this above, but when there's not enough staff, the current staff have to pick up the slack. The question to ask is, why are practices and hospitals understaffed? Lots of reasons, but one of the main reasons is money. The business folks running the hospital business are under the gun to perform financially and produce a profit, yet they often have insurmountable problems to overcome if they want to turn a profit. One thing they can do, and do it all the time, is cut staff to the point where the nurses who stay are able to handle the load.

If you think this isn't calculated, think again! Worker productivity is a highly refined industry skill set and if you knew the mechanisms of thought that go into it, you'd be highly offended. So...let me actually create a little offense on this and describe a hypothetical scenario just so you can understand how these managers and businesspeople are thinking in a medical business setting.

Manager: How do we maximize productivity and save money?

Consultant: Let's see, how productive are your current employees?

Manager: We calculate that our staff have about 75% work engagement that produces revenue for the hospital. 25% spent on non-essential non-revenue producing activities.

Consultant: So, what you're telling me is that out of ever 4 employees you have one extra that doesn't need to be there.

Manager: Well, I suppose, but we're already short staffed.

Consultant: You're not short staffed you just don't have 100% work engagement from the staff you do have.

Manager: We can't make them work at 100% capacity on revenue producing activities, they would revolt or burn out.

Consultant: It all depends on how it's presented.

Manager: OK, I'm listening

Consultant: You have to appeal to their emotional side to convince them to work harder, but you also have to boil the frog in the process. (the reference to boiling a frog means that if you through a frog in hot water it will jump out, but if you slowly increase the temperature it won't notice and it will eventually die without trying jump out, hence, that's how you boil a frog.)

Manager: Keep going

Consultant: Appeal to the staff that you are short staffed and that you can't afford to bring on more staff. Then appeal to them that the true purpose of their work is to care for the patient, (that's always the appeal in medicine when you're try to get more work out of staff), let's use the concept of the patient to overcome objections about pay and benefits because you have a moral compass on caring for patients.) Then explain that "we" includes the hospital and also includes patients, making them associate patients with the hospital so they will believe that their altruistic efforts to work harder can be accomplished by serving the hospital, not just the individual patient in a bed. Then explain the need to do the best we can to serve the patients (aka hospital entity) with the staff we do have.

Manager: OK, so how do we implement this?

Consultant: Start by not replacing staff after they quit or leave, that is a natural process for the remaining staff to pick up the slack, they will feel an obligation to cover the duties of the other staff member that left "until they are replaced" for the purpose of serving the patients with the best care. BUT you don't replace them, you instead test the waters to see how well the remaining staff can integrate and handle the duties of the former worker who left. If one staff member complains about picking up too much of the other staff members work you simple delegate some of that work out, now that remaining staff member feels heard and the new staff member that picked up some of those extra duties is made to feel like they are supporting this other staff member in their overload of work. Now you are engaging their moral drive for patient care and channeling it toward your hospital business entity, and you are engaging the natural family support instinct to support the other staff.

Manager: Wow! That's an amazing way to handle that! How do you know they will handle it this way?

Consultant: Because they are part of a "family", a team that supports each other for the purpose of caring for sick patients which is an emotionally satisfying effort. You have to use the term family to describe the employee group so that people will feel an emotional obligation to step up and help. There's less room for slacking when there's not enough staff members, and nobody wants to let down a family member or see patients suffer, and now you have subtly increased efficiency of the staff and utilized their emotional connection to other staff members as a way to "encourage" them to work harder and produce more revenue generating activity.

Manager: OK, so let's map out a plan of action on this!

Manager is then going to create a scenario where the hospital will become more profitable, and the management and corporate leadership will likely reward that manager with bonuses and perks for having increased margins and profitability.

This is a hypothetical scenario, but it draws from a lot of real life examples I've read about studies and actually heard people describe and use in real medical businesses I've worked with. I even had one HR director in one of my companies talk about how not re-hiring a position and expecting the remaining staff to pick up the load as commonly understood HR tactic for increasing worker productivity.

Now it makes so much more sense why medical staff burn out so often! They don't realize how they are being stressed intentionally to increase productivity until they just give up altogether and quit. Actually, you want to read about some real twisted manager employee manipulation tactics for increasing worker productivity without increasing labor spend, look up the Wal Mart middle management training tactics. They probably don't openly publish those, but there are plenty of news articles about this that describe things like emotionally manipulating employees to work off the clock to finish things, while using guilt, shame, embarrassment, fear, and all sorts of other tactics. The more of that kind of activity that exists in the workplace the further and further they will push people to be unhappy and leave. Most employees aren't going to express their genuine internal feelings about why they are unhappy or tell those things to a manager who they already believe is using personal information and personal interactions with them to abuse the situation to get the employee to work harder, the employee will just quit rather than talk about it, so the managers never really know why they keep failing at this.

I can't say it loud enough, you avoid ALL these problems when you have your own business and you're an independent contractor.

Sure, there are a lot of other things to worry about, but it all changes when you are in control of your own operation. Your internal drive is entirely different when the work you're doing is your own!

3. **Lack of Autonomy**

I think you already know how this is overcome, but like I just described, you're in control of "most" of your work and schedule. I put most in parentheses because you're still operating under a provider's orders and following a treatment plan so you can't just do a bunch of extra stuff that you haven't been approved for, but you likely already know this, but I just wanted to point this out.

Autonomy DOES come into play in how you execute on the treatment plan orders. The provider is ordering a treatment plan for the patient that is an 8-week plan with two treatments a week. How you go about that is up to you and the patient, but you have the autonomy to set that schedule with the patient.

Regarding autonomy of your schedule. You set your schedule, but you still want to accommodate patients' needs so you'll work with them, but that conversation is between you and the patient not between you and a manager. So, the idea of going the extra mile is actually a welcome concept when you're working out the best schedule for that patient and for yourself. Also, you can simply not accept that patient if you can't accommodate them. It's not a matter of a manager telling you you must take them and also work into the evening to accommodate them; you just get to decide you can't fit them into your schedule and you move on with a patient load you can handle. Simple as that!

4. **Poor Work-Life Balance**

Well, I think I covered the work-life balance concept above, but since we're on that, work-life balance changes drastically when you own your own business and control your own schedule. You can control how much you do or don't do!

What's also really cool is that if you want to increase your income for a period of time, you can simply opt to take more patients for a while, earn the extra income, and then cut back. You can also cut back to half-time or quarter-time if your income is enough to cover your needs and satisfy your lifestyle. Some nurses are going to make over $20k a month and some are going to make $5-6k and be just fine because that income is reflected in how much time they spent seeing patients. You control that.

Need to take a break for a week for vacation? Well, you can let your patients know ahead of time that you're taking a break and work that out, or you could hand them over to another nurse while you're gone, people like extra money, so that may be easy, OR you could consider expanding your operation, because it is your operation, and brining in more people to work for you in a similar model, but within your entity. I'll talk about this in the last section on expanding your business an making a million a year or more.

5. Limited Career Advancement

Career advancement?!? What's that again? You own your own damn business and you're advanced as it gets! Nobody else to report to in your own business but you!

Keep in mind that your patients are your clients. So...you can still get fired from seeing them, or you can fire them if you aren't comfortable seeing them, so just remember that being the top dog in your company doesn't mean you can just disregard everyone else. You're still serving patients in need, and they are depending on you to deliver care to them for pain relief, and you need to do that to make money for yourself, so you still have some element of someone to deal with. But this is present in all positions that deal with people. There's always someone higher to report to. When you're the business owner you report to your clients and customers, because you need them. When you are an employee you report to your boss, because they are the person in control of keeping your paycheck rolling.

Back to career advancement, there are many ways to grow your business and I'm going to share those with you, but just know that you are already at the top of your company when it's your own company, so if there was ever a career boosting action you could take, this is the action!

6. **Inadequate Compensation**

   How about a $1,000,000 a year? Yeah, I think you can call that adequate compensation. On that note I do want to point out that there are a few things to do in your business to get to that level of take-home pay for yourself, but it's absolutely within reach once you get started, so keep that in mind, you absolutely have the ability to make a million dollars a year or more by owning and operating you our mobile pain treatment business.

7. **Lack of Recognition and Appreciation**

   I can't stress enough how grateful your patients are going to be! It truly is a life altering line of work and I've seen hundreds of employees and staff who had never experienced what it was like to be truly appreciated by their patients and their work environment!

   Let's outline all the parties who are going to be extremely grateful for your work and who may confront you with tears in their eyes of gratitude for your work. You probably think I'm embellishing this to get you excited, but after you get started, you'll know exactly what I'm talking about:

Patients – Your patients are going to have their lives changed for the better and they are going to thank you profusely for bringing life back to their life. Most patients are in such pain that walking around the house creates a dangerous level of anxiety and increased blood pressure just knowing that they are about to endure pain just going to the bathroom or walking to the kitchen. When they are relieved of pain and skipping around the house, they are going to be extremely grateful to you. That kind of recognition is the ultimate reward. Side note here: In one of my practices I had a nurse tell me that she'd never experienced patients having an upward trajectory in health and life. All the patients she'd worked with in career had only experienced downward trajectories. Internal Medicine and Pain Management will admit that the continual flow of health for their patients is downward. They are effectively managing the downward spiral of health and trying to prevent as much damage as possible along the way. That's all they can do. Neurofunctional Pain Management changes the entire playing field. People get better and improve their health and actually get their life back! Trust me, you'll see this firsthand yourself.

Patients Families – Their family members are going to likely hug you and cry with you about how grateful they are for you treating their family member and getting them out of pain. How many spouses have cried in our offices with our staff members, tears of joy, over their spouse getting out of pain. What a wonderful feeling it is to be the nurse that is helping them do this! It's truly a life changing line of work, and I'm talking about the life changing part being you. You're going to love your job again; you'll be able to realize those dreams you had while in nursing school of caring for the sick and helping them get better and feeling like you made a difference. The medical field likely has beaten those dreams out of you by now, but they are still available, and they will be yours! Go and live that dream and be happy in your work!

The Pain Doctor - If there is a pain specialist involved, they'll be really happy about the pain relief result, and that it doesn't require medications. They may still be a procedure centered pain doctors or office, but they'll ultimately be happy about the program working in a mobile setting where they likely wouldn't be able to help the patient much.

Primary Care Providers - Primary care providers are usually surprised by the improvement and the pain relief. It's very common for patients to reduce meds or get off meds as a result of the program. In fact, here are some of the surprising benefits of the program that would appeal to a patient's primary care doctor. The primary benefit most patients report is improved sleep and sleeping through the night. This is a huge one! Here are the others, reduced stress and anxiety related to chronic pain, improved cardiovascular function and blood pressure improvement, improved respiratory function including increased VO2 max and breathing, reduced local inflammation and reduced systemic inflammation, increased physical activity, improved diet and eating habits, and reduction in a range of medications. So, you might be asking, how does all this stuff happen with just this treatment? Getting out of pain produces a whole cascade of benefits, and the electrical treatment actually stimulates a range of neurotransmitters that are responsible for a lot of overall health improvements.

Regarding all the health benefits of the program, I've seen doctors be completely surprised by the unexpected health benefits and the requests to get off medications. One doctor started calling me about how all these patients on our program started having regular health blood pressure and he wanted to know what was going on, in a good way! So, there are a lot of great supplemental benefits to the program beyond just getting out of pain, as if pain relief wasn't enough already!

8. **Physical Demands and Health Risks**

This is the one thing that can still factor into this equation. You still need to be physically able to get around and work with patients. It's not the same as the physically demanding environment of a hospital where you might be moving patients around and such. You'll need to carry a few supplies, and the electrical device isn't too bad to tote around, but you still have to go in and out of houses, up and down stairs, and do some basic physical activities like that.

Keep in mind that the Get to Have to equation factors in here as well. It's not as hard when it's your own business and you love what you do. So, despite the physical aspect of this job, it's going to be much more enjoyable work when it's your own choice to do it.

Health risks could still be considered a problem, as some people may be sick in other ways, but keep in mind that as your own business you can decide who all you're going to treat and you can decided not to accept a patient that doesn't meet your own personal safety requirements and refusing to accept them won't require you to explain yourself to management or to fill out forms and such.

9. **Administrative Burden**

Hahaha, I think we got this one covered! You are your own supervisor and administrator so try not to be too hard on yourself!

I suppose there are always people to report to in any scenario, but at least in this scenario the people you're reporting to are not hanging on your every move and breathing over your shoulder. The people you report to in this program are likely going to be the medical office who ordered the treatment program, and likely you'll have very little correspondence with them as they are not going to be involved in the daily treatment program you're carrying out. You will send in the basic notes and such for the treatment event that day so the office can conduct billing, and you may need to chat with the office or doctor about patients occasionally, but it's nothing like most nurses are used to with a half dozen layers of leadership over you all requesting a range of updates and details about everything you did, are doing, and will do in a given shift.

10. Moral Distress

Again, I think this concept is a moot point in regard to your work as a mobile pain treatment nurse. In the common complaint section nurses mentioned the moral distress came from not being able to offer the care needed and having moral stress over it. I think that's a distant memory when you're operating this program and you're providing all the benefit we described above. So, not only do you not have to deal with negative moral stress, but you're also dealing with positive moral relief that you are able to give patients what they need to get better. It's a moral morale boost!

OK, so now you have a much better understanding of all the benefits of doing this. I'm also sure you've already started to imagine that it's much more than just a business to make money, it's a whole new outlook on your career as a nurse, and you have the ability to do great things and impact people's lives for the better!

I'd also like to point out that many of your patients will seek out a treatment program every year, so you'll likely get to know them and become friends with them and their families over time. I want to recap some of the unexpected benefits of the program, the stuff you may not be aware of or thinking about but are definitely real and part of this whole process.

Unexpected benefits of this program: Patients don't just experience pain relief; they have a whole range of health benefits that occur with this treatment program, and you'll get to see these changes. Improved sleep, reduced stress, improved behavioral health issues like improvements in depression and anxiety as a result of reduced pain and the systemic release of neurotransmitters that assist in this category of health, increased respiratory activity, improved cardiovascular function, increased physical activity, increased outlook on life, reduced medications, improved relationships with family and loved ones, and in some cases a regaining of quality-of-life functions. Side note: I've seen patients be able to get their drivers license reinstated after they got out of pain and proved they were better, so that's something you just don't think about! There are many more possible improvements I can't think of at this moment, but I'm sure people will remind me.

Literally changing lives for the better: Once people are out of pain their quality of life is just better all around. You'll see this happen firsthand and you'll be credited with making I possible, so that's a huge win for nurse and patient!

Offering hope where it didn't exist: I believe in hope, and I know that when people actually succeed in getting out of pain after having a chronic pain condition for decades, that their outlook on life is restored, their hope is restored. Side note: In one office a patient actually wrote a thank you card to our nurse in the office and told her that she had given him much more than just pain relief, she had given him hope. I think that says all I can say about hope.

Strengthening families and relationships: If you've ever been around a chronic pain patient, you'll know they are not easy to be around. Sometimes the constant complaining or the constant reminders to everyone that they are uncomfortable, or in pain, or unable to engage in a family activity make it really hard to have a quality relationship with that person. Also, I've talked to several people who claim that grandma or grandpa just completely changed when they got put on opioids for their pain. The grandparents were also sad that they felt the need to take an opioid pill before company comes over so they can at least be out of pain while they had visitors, but instead were dealing with the effects of being on drugs while trying to enjoy time with family. What a hard situation to be in, and what a sad state of life to be on pain meds while trying to spend quality time with family.

That said, getting people out of pain the healthy way without medications produces substantially better social experiences and the ability to strengthen your family and social relationships. If your parents or grandparents are out of pain and off medications for pain and can walk around freely without pain, imagine how much happier they will be and all the rest of your friends and family will be.

One other aspect is that of marriages and relationships. I'm no marriage expert, but I have known that chronic pain can create an extremely difficult marriage environment. I know one couple who were married for decades and when the husband entered into a state of chronic pain and ended up on medications, he changed and his wife tried to make it work, but after a while she could no longer stand the situation. Again, I'm no expert on relationships, but nobody wants to be in a relationship where constant drug use is required to just relieve the pain. Getting patients out of pain without medications can literally change the outcome of their lives and relationships, so I hope all of you reading this understand that there's so much more to what you're doing than just treating people for pain.

Chapter 6

The business of operating a mobile pain treatment program

Alright! Here's the scoop on how this works as a business! I'm going to guide you through all the details so you can understand how to build your own operation. Let's dive in!

1) **Operating your own entity under a medical director:**

   You're operating as an independent contractor nurse, but you still need a medical director to perform work on patients and be generally cleared for activity. A medical director doesn't have to be "in business" with you, they just need to be medically responsible for what you're doing. In this program the treatments are super simple and very safe. There are hardly any contraindications, you'll go through those in training, and most doctors would be fine being a medical director. The hard part is that most doctors want the same payment to be a medical director for one nurse as the would for a small company, so I have created a platform model for this with my company RELATYV. We have a medical director in each state who is aware of what we do and approves of our activity and is willing to be the director over the state for all our nurses and technicians. This will allow you to operate independently like you're hoping and still be covered affordably. The platform model wins the day because you'd pay way more for a medical director on your own.

2) **Your own insurances:**

Yes, you will need your own malpractice, but for a nurse or other non-provider medical professional, malpractice is very inexpensive because they know you are operating under the direction of a medical director and you're only performing services that a provider has requested, so I've typically seen malpractice for RNs ranging from $250-350/year. YES, that's per year. It's really not that bad. Now you'll need some general business liability insurance to cover yourself and your equipment in case of theft or damage. You definitely want this because you just never know what could happen and the last think you want is the unexpected slapping you in the face right when your business is taking off! Equipment and general liability for a small business like this is usually only a few hundred a year. Not too bad either. You could likely get all your insurance coverage for $500-600 a year and that's a steal compared to what other businesses pay, and what the doctors are paying for their own malpractice. I don't even want to speculate; just know you've got it made at only a few hundred a year!

3) **Ancillary services details, stark law and other details:**

There are several ways to work as an independent service provider to medical offices. My favorite way is that of an ancillary service provider! This is a special type of relationship where you offer a special medical service to a doctor or medical practice for the purpose of billing Medicare and commercials payers for that service. If your service isn't billable work, then you likely don't need an ancillary service agreement in most cases. In this case, we would want an ancillary service agreement because Neurofunctional Pain Management is all billable. In case you haven't heard of the Stark Law, this is a law put in place to keep doctors from being incentivized to perform unnecessary or excessive medical services. I'll quote Google here for you so can get a succinct description. "The

Stark law, also known as the Physician Self-Referral Law, is a federal civil law that limits the financial relationships between physicians and entities that provide "designated health services" (DHS). The law prohibits physicians from referring patients to receive DHS from entities with which they or an immediate family member have a financial relationship, unless an exception applies. DHS include services like physical and occupational therapies, radiology services, and inpatient hospital services. Financial relationships include ownership, investment interests, and compensation arrangements." (Google AI Response). I would like to add to this that a physician can absolutely refer to an entity in which they have a financial interest as long as they comply with a few rules about it and it's disclosed to anyone they refer. I suppose asking Google won't give you all the answers, but at the very least you have an idea of what this is. I also heard from several experts that Stark Law was triggered by the relationship of physicians and various labs that were paying physicians to send in samples.

What this means is that this law is trying to stop doctors from doing things just to make money, or the term unduly incentivizing physicians to perform services really makes this easy to understand. However, doctors can't possibly do everything themselves so they have to refer patients out for almost everything the doctor can't handle in house, as you can see from the list above. So, where does that leave you with offering your services? It's as simple as having the right paperwork in place with the office!

You can operate in a safe realm of the Stark Law called the Safe Harbor section. This spells out the relationship that is allowed for doctors to make a financial profit on work performed for their practice, like I mentioned above, billable services. Here's a quick Google definition of the safe harbor section. "The Stark Law's safe harbor provisions define payment and business practices that are not considered kickbacks, bribes, or rebates that may unlawfully induce payment from Medicare or Medicaid programs. These provisions also specify allowable financial and referral relationships between physicians and other providers and suppliers." (Google AI Response). So, there you have it! You can perform billable services for doctors with the right paperwork in place. It can be complex, and I'm not an attorney so I can't give you any legal advice except that if you want to do this on your own, you will want an attorney to review your paperwork.

I've owned and operated ancillary services companies for about a decade now and I've had the same general paperwork I've used that has passed the sniff test with dozens and dozens of medical offices and their attorneys so I'm pretty happy with my ancillary services contract, but I still have an attorney take a look every now and then to make sure I'm still good. Also, the service models can change a bit for what you're doing over time, so it doesn't hurt to have it reviewed occasionally. Though it does hurt to pay for that review. This is why I'm promoting the idea that you operate your new mobile pain treatment business within my platform, so you'll have this coverage already in place, because my company has these agreements with all the offices we work with, so any nurse I bring into my platform is covered! So, one more aspect of value I'm trying to offer to help you be successful!

4) Qualifications for operating equipment and training credentials:

I work with the best equipment manufacturer in this space who owns the patent on the high-pulse technology needed to produce the pain relief effect and all the other health benefits that result from using the right electrical therapy. This is all put together in a package that can easily be financed with any bank or equipment financing group. Most financial institutions love medical professionals and are almost blinded by the titles in my opinion. A doctor graduating from medical school can get huge lines of credit just because of the title. They also get special home purchasing privileges like now having their student loans count against them in the mortgage process. I talked to an actual underwriter about this once, and from what I can tell, banks are just blinded by credentials and willing to throw money at titles. They used to do this with attorneys as well, but I don't think it's a easy as it used to be for them, but doctors still walk into the bank and they roll out the red carpet!

All that said, I'm really just trying to express that there is a bit of positive favoritism in the financing world toward medical professionals. So, it should be easier to get financing on a smaller piece of equipment than you might expect. You'll then need to go through training. Training isn't difficult at all. I have trained dozens of people myself in a couple of hours and then it's just a little practice. My nurse training team can get you trained on the equipment via a zoom session, so you don't even have to travel. You can even see your first patients and have the training nurse on a zoom chat to assist if needed, but you'll be able to practice a few times before your first patient and then you're never looking back!

Who can operate this machine? Any medical staff member who would be able to touch patients in an office setting is allowed to use this medical device under medical supervision. Here's the basic list; RN, CNA, LPN, LVN, EMT, OTA, CA, MA, and I'm sure I'm missing a few others, but if your certification or license allows to help/handle/touch patients in a medical setting you're good to go on handling this equipment and treating patients.

The IV portion of the program would need to be conducted by RNs and we do run into specific regulations at the state level regarding nurses offering IVs in homes, but this is all a little more streamlined when its operating through a doctor's office ordering care on patients as an ancillary service. Another reason I like to operate this way.

Also, any medical person I've listed above can perform the health coaching that goes with our program, they will just need to complete a little training on health coaching because it's not just something you guess at or wing on the spot. Health coaching is a reimbursable activity so it has to be performed properly and documented, but anyone can do it and it adds to the total value of the program and the health of the patient so it's a win-win for everyone!

5) **Medicare and commercial coverage and the pay cycle and how you get paid:**

OK, so now you see why the ancillary concept is so important because you can't just willy nilly provide billable medical services to a physician or medical practice without the proper paperwork in place. This also means that if services are covered by Medicare and commercial payers you should not have a hard time getting a full schedule! Particularly in the field of chronic pain management. Like I mentioned above, there are around 50 million people in the US suffering with a chronic pain condition, so that is a lot of potential for you to keep a full schedule. One of the problems with most areas and rural areas is access to a provider, or access to a provider who is able to do something besides pain medications. Neurofunctional Pain Management is a game-changer in the ability to offer something safe to patients. What you're offering here is more than just a pain treatment, it's literally saving lives. Here's just one example. We are all familiar with fall risk and hospitalization and subsequent death from complications. Many people have died from simply losing balance over dealing with a chronic pain issue and been hospitalized and then passed away in the hospital as a result of the fall injury. I once wrote a paper on this, and I focused on the reasons for the falls. They always identify balance as one of the primary reasons, and many patients will tell interviewers that they lost balance and fell, but what you don't see a whole lot of is the reason for losing balance. In more cases than we might imagine, it's the patient shifting their weight because of pain and then losing their balance. It's much more common than we expect. With that in mind, you truly are preventing patients from going down this path and saving lives in that sense. Also, avoiding medications and opiates is another way you could be saving lives with this work. The point of this is to discuss Medicare reimbursement and the primary demographic of patients needing this program, Medicare age patients with chronic pain.

Here's how you get paid in this ancillary model. If you are on your own, then you would structure a payment agreement with your doctor or practice that you're performing services for. This can be a percentage of the reimbursement created from the work you perform or a flat fee. You'll hear some people say percents aren't compliant and that flat fees are better, but this isn't the case. You can arrange percent deals and maintain all the steps to be compliant. Sure, flat rates are easier, but doctors have a harder time with flat rates unless your rates are substantially lower than the reimbursement, so the doctor doesn't have to take too much risk of loss or delay on reimbursement. Typically, if you are structuring a percent model, you're at the mercy of the reimbursement revenue cycle which is a flywheel that starts spinning and spinning, with payments taking weeks to months to process and you just have to wait. You're also at the mercy of the billing service the doctor uses. It could be in-house or a third-party billing service. Not sure I can say which is better I've seen both work and both fail so ideally you want to talk to your doctor group you're working with about their billing. Remember, you're at the mercy of reimbursement to the doctor's office so anything that does wrong with that and you're on the hook as well, good or bad. This might make you think, OK I'll do a flat rate, but most doctors and practices are wise to this as well and they'll require you to wait on reimbursement before being paid, or they just won't do a deal with you at all. So flat rate doesn't guarantee payment for you. Either way, after you perform services, you can expect a doctor's office to only reconcile their billing and pay out once a month. You should also expect that they are only going to pay out on what's been collected, not what's been billed and is still pending. So just bear that in mind as you conduct operations.

All this confusion over the billing process is another reason why I think working though our platform is ideal! We arrange all the ancillary agreements with providers. We work with them on the billing process, and we do our reconciliation with them all each month. Our provider groups pay our company a negotiated rate for service, my company takes a small booking fee for managing the whole process, and the rest is paid to the nurse for services performed. This is how nurses get paid in our system. Pretty easy and we take all the stress out of working with doctors' offices. There's strength in numbers, and if you're by yourself you don't have a lot of firepower to argue with a doctor or practice over pretty much anything, but when you're part of our larger group we are bringing so much value to the doctor or practice that they don't want to upset our apple cart. All we have to do is shift our patient flow to another provider group if the one we're working with is playing games on paying their invoices. We tell all of them that the most valuable aspect of our relationship and partnership with a medical group is the timely payment of our invoices for services performed because we pay the nurses who do all the work and they are not likely to go out and do work under a particular doctor's office if they know that office will delay payments and argue about things all the time. The larger the business volume for the doctor the more risk there is in losing us as a service, but we all play nice and we all need each other and we all know it, so I don't really see much of this happening. I have had offices who intentionally delayed payment only to find out they had much bigger problems going on inside their practice, so it really does matter that you find a good physician or practice to work with. We do this for you and our providers know the value our service is bringing, so we are all in alignment!

6) **Marketing and patient acquisition:**

Patient flow is the most important aspect of your business. All the other stuff is just business structure, the patient is your actual client that generates your income. I know it's vulgar to associate patients with dollar amounts, but patients are how you get paid, so they are clients and you need to treat them like a valuable client, not just "another patient you have to deal with" like you may feel when working in a regular W2 position in a busy office where you don't have to care if the work you do generates revenue because you get paid the same regardless. This is your business now and each patient is your client, and they may stay your client for decades and get treatment on a regular basis from you. They also refer to new clients/patients, so this is how you build your business!

I say all this because you need patients and if you don't have a plan for patients, you don't have much of a business. You'll get a few patients from the office you're running your billing through, but they may not use you to your full capacity. Some offices may fill you up fast. This is why I always promote my RELATYV platform because we are able to drive patient flow in many ways and get your schedule filled and keep it filled! So, whether you are on your own, or working with my platform, your key objective for business success is patient flow!

7) The Million Dollar Nurse - Expanding and growing your business:

OK, so now you know all this info above and you might be asking the question, the title of the book says Million Dollar Nurses, so how does that work for me? Great question and I have a great answer! Being an independent contractor means you are operating as a small business entity. You have the ability to treat your entity like a regular business that can grow and expand. So, now that you have experience in your business activities and treating patients, you can look at how to expand your own services within your business. Regarding my platform, I don't hire individual nurses as 1099 contractors, I contract with an entity as a 1099 contractor that happens to be owned by you, the nurse who is performing services. When we pay out the earnings to a nurse, we are actually paying that to your entity, not you individually as a person. This means that if you expand your entity to include more people, then your entity would get paid for all the work that was generated under that entity. What we are talking about here is expanding your operation so that you can achieve a million dollars a year in take-home revenue for yourself.

One of the easiest things you can do is add an MA or CNA to your team. They are eligible to operate the electrical equipment on their own and they can handle the visits that pay less because there is no IV or other activity on those days, just the electrical treatment event. An MA or CNA is used to getting paid a certain amount that usually isn't that impressive for them. You could bring them into your team, have them doing treatments just like you, and they would likely be very happy with even half the revenue they generate for your entity.

Let's conduct an example really quick. Let's assume you have a full schedule of patients, which for a mobile treatment program is about 6 treatments a day, 5 days a week, and let's assume you are working

52 weeks a year. I know people take time off, but I'm just showing you what's possible here.

Neurofunctional Pain Management consists of two treatments a week, one electrical treatment and one electrical with IV combined treatment. The difference in reimbursement between is enough to make it work hiring someone else to cover the simpler treatment for you.

Hypothetical example of how to build your team
$120 Electrical only treatment revenue
$200 Electrical and IV combined revenue

You hire an MA to work for you and do all the electrical only treatments for you. Remember that you're really only able to handle about 30 events a week, so let's assume a full schedule of 30 electrical events a week conducted by your MA

$120x30 = $3600/week or $187, 200/year

Your MA is perfectly happy and actually very excited to earn less than half that even paying for their own car and travel. Let's call this $80,000 a year to your MA. You know any other MA's making $80,000 a year? This is more than twice what the average MA makes, so they are likely going to be really excited about this, same with a CNA.

Now, you as the nurse are free to do all the combo treatment events that pay more, $200/event. $200 x 30 = $6000/week or $312,000/year for your higher dollar events that you cover. Now add the difference you kept from your MA's work $107,200 and you have a total of $419,000 a year gross net for yourself.

You're nearly halfway to that million dollar a year mark. So, think you can convince a couple of your nurse friends to come on board with your small business and get paid much better than they would elsewhere and work with someone they like being around? Well, now you can see how doing this same model with a couple more nurses and MA's will tip you over the million a year mark.

You'll want to express the value you bring to the table by them joining you, such as paying for their equipment and supplies, so they have no out of pocket expenses. The equipment is a bit of an expense, so if you're paying for that, it can be enough to convince a lot of people to work in your business. In fact, I have a sponsor program in place so that any nurses who are trying to build out their work group within their business, we'll deliver nurses to them who may not be able to purchase their own equipment but would love to do this. If you bought the equipment package, they'd likely be willing to come into your group and make far less than they would on their own, but don't have to put up any money for equipment and supplies, so it's a win-win for both of you.

You know what some people think is an amazing perk that's pretty affordable and could probably convince a nurse to come on board? A car stipend and a food stipend! Super affordable perks you can offer them as 1099 employees in your new business that will help convince them to come on board.

Also, don't forget that you are doing great things for patients and remember this phrase because it's so true in this scenario. "You'll fall back in love with nursing all over again!" Will Bozeman. Yes, I just quoted myself, but I truly believe the work you're doing is going to change your life and the lives of all your patients. So don't forget to explain that this is more than just a job or income, it's making a difference and all your colleagues who want to work with you will love this!

Chapter 7

RELATYV Mobile Pain Treatment Platform

The RELATYV Mobile Pain Treatment Platform is the platform I built to accommodate this entire program. It functions a lot like an Airbnb model where you make yourself available as a nurse, and we can then start driving patients to you and fill up your schedule to your liking. We also seek out all the physician and medical practice relationships, so we are covering all the hard parts of getting this going.

All about the benefits of using a platform to grow your business.

We want to help you build your business and grow it into a million-dollar income for you! There's no reason why you can't make a million dollars a year doing work you love and changing people's lives. "You can have anything you want in this life if you help enough people get what they want." This is a famous quote from Zig Zigler the motivational speaker. He's absolutely correct in this case. People want to get out of pain, and they want their lives back. You are giving them what they want and if you do that enough you'll get what you want, excellent income, freedom in your work, respect from your friend's family and community, and a sense of fulfillment that you're doing something productive and useful for people in need. Like I tell everyone, you'll fall back in love with nursing all over again!

The benefits of using a platform like RELATYV to build your business are probably obvious to many of you, but not so obvious to others. I'll list out some of the benefits here, but first I want to point out that you can absolutely do this yourself if you really wanted to and not use my platform. So, just know that what I'm telling you is my opinion on why the platform is useful, but you could definitely go it alone if you wanted.

I want to list these in order of importance (in my opinion of importance)

1) **Patient flow:** You have to have this! It is your actual business. No patients, no business. A platform is designed to fill you up with patients and keep you as busy as you want. This is also a result of scale and branding that the platform brings.

2) **Physician relationships:** You probably have these relationships, BUT that does not mean they'll engage you as an ancillary service. Some doctors just don't do those kinds of deals so having that pre-arranged is really convenient for you to just get started.

3) **Compliance:** You will need to operate compliantly, and ancillary programs operate within the Stark Law as I described above, so knowing you're in the compliance zone is great. If you're on your own, you'll need to work with an attorney on this.

4) **Protocol and treatment model:** I created Neurofunctional Pain Management years ago and have refined this treatment model. Sure, it could be copied, but my operation has it nailed down, so you don't have to re-create that.

5) **Billing and coding for Physician Partners:** So even if you replicate the treatment protocol, you still have to know how to bill it properly. That is a whole different thing from just copying it. I've seen offices fumble this all over the field. If you're offering your services as an ancillary service provider, you'll need to be able to connect

the billing office with the resources and expertise they need to bill this properly.

6) **Equipment package and training:** We have the equipment package all put together so make this a convenient way to launch your business. Contact me about an equipment package and we'll get you going!

7) **Medical director:** Sure, any medical provider can be your director, but they usually charge you more than you need for this. My platform offers this at a substantially reduced rate. Again, it's a matter of scale for us, so we can reduce costs.

8) **Community of colleagues:** This could be argued to be at the top of the list. This community of colleagues' aspect is really a big part of the operation. Even operating as your own business, you can still collaborate with colleagues in the same situation as you. Competition amongst each other, you might ask? Sure, there could be a little, but remember that 15 patients is a full load of patients for you if you're treating them on the regular cycle, so you can't really dominate an area and take away all the patients from your competitors. There are literally millions of patients who need this, and they'll need this on a regular basis year after year. The competition aspect could be more involved in recruiting other nurses and techs to work under you, but that's just part of business in general. The ability to chat with all the other nurses out there and learn about what they are doing and how they are succeeding is a huge benefit to being successful!

I'm sure I'm missing a few benefits, and I hope you will point those out for me so I can update the book for next time. A platform really can launch you straight into action and success. So I promote the platform, yet I fully respect a nurse's desire to do this on their own. I'll do the best I can to help you and point you in the right direction!

Taking your first step in launching your own business.

So, here's the big leap, the first step in launching your own business and starting your path to making a million a year with your own mobile pain treatment business. I'll list these out for you, and it will make all this really easy to follow:

1) Create your entity: If you already have an entity, great, you're good to go and skip this. Every state has a super easy way to create an LLC on your own and usually its really cheap. If you aren't sure how to do it, just ask someone. Chances are a ton of people know exactly what to do in your state. In Arizona I can go to the Arizona Corporation Commission website, click on start a new business, select the type of business like LLC, then enter my information like the name of the business I'm choosing, and a few other details, then I pay the fee of $35 and I'm good to go! They'll let me know when it's live via email and I can just go in and see that it's active by doing an entity name search and seeing it as live or active. Super easy!

2) Employer Identification Number EIN or Tax Identification Number TIN: This is the IRS number attached to your business. You'll need this to open a business bank account. You can knock this out in literally 2 min on the IRS website and it's sooo easy, so don't be afraid of this. https://sa.www4.irs.gov/modiein/individual/index.jsp. This is the direct link to the application on the IRS website, but you can Google it and just follow the clicks to apply now until you get to the application. Don't fall for the sponsored ads for an EIN that will pop up on the Google search. There are lot of companies hoping you'll click on them thinking they are the official site, and they'll try to charge you something, but IRS.gov is the main domain and getting an EIN is free, so if it don't say IRS.gov in your link it ain't the right place. Knock this out and it's super easy to do at the same time as you apply for your LLC. Two things that make you an official business and you knocked them out in like five min!!!

3) Business bank account: Everyone's bank is different, but I can open a business bank account on my bank app in about 5 min. Super easy and I have a separate business bank account for each business I operate, and I have about a dozen businesses I own. If you can knock this out online, great, if you have to go into your bank, they'll take care of you, because they are excited about business accounts, so you may get a little of the royal treatment! I used to get offered snacks and such while I waited because they like business owners. Never had them offer me a snack for waiting in line to do anything else. They may require your LLC to be live before allowing the account to be formed. Bank rules are more strict that a couple decades ago so they jump through more protection hoops, but it's still super easy to do this. Then you'll have a business account.

4) Equipment package: These previous three items above apply to any new business venture, but this one is specific to the mobile pain treatment program. You'll need the proper equipment for this. My company works directly with the manufacturer and the financing group to make sure we get the nurses a full equipment package that gets them up and running. This typically includes the electroanalgesia machine, the initial batch of IV supplies and other basic supplies. I was inclined to list the package cost here, but it can change based on market availability and global demand for equipment, so I don't want to quote it here, but I'm happy to discuss it with anyone wanting to move forward. Luckily, most people are able to finance this and get started with a payment that is only a few hundred dollars a month. In some areas of the country the income potential for a single person is well over $200k and if you wanted to crank out the work you could put in more work and more time. It's all up to you, but keep in mind that you can hire more of your own staff and purchase equipment for them to keep growing and expanding your services. That's the path to a million dollars a year like I discussed above.

You CAN do this!!!

There's so much opportunity and abundance out there! I realize there may be a million reasons not to do this, but I'm trying to help you see that there are also potentially a million reasons a year to do this!

Launching your own business and taking control of your financial life, your personal schedule, your drive and ambition, and your life in general seems overwhelming for some people. I agree it can be a lot to do all at once, but you can take the steps to get there in manageable ways. You don't have to quit your day job and jump into owning your own mobile pain treatment operation overnight. You can start as a part time operation and build it up. You can manage the risk and make this work in a less risky way. I told the story of my Amazon store above for this very purpose, to show you that you can start your own venture and build your own business while you are still working for a wage to pay the bills! It's possible and I know you have the ability to do this.

Let me and my team help you do this!

Reach out to me and I'll get you started and help you build this business that changes your life forever.

will@relatyv.com
www.willbozeman.com
www.relatyv.com

One day you'll be in a group photo of all the Million Dollar Nurses from around the nation who took this leap and changed their life for the better, and genuinely improved the lives of everyone you served along the way.

Contact me and let's get you started!

Fall back in love with nursing all over again!

Join the ranks of the Million Dollar Nurses!

About the Author

Will Bozeman is a healthcare executive, innovator, entrepreneur, inventor, author, and writer with a wide range of experience in the medical field. Wil has multiple degrees in a variety of subjects that give depth to his capability as an entrepreneur and his ability to operate as an innovative healthcare executive. Will has attended medical school in Alabama and holds an associate degree in electrical technology, two undergraduate degrees in biotechnology and archeology, and an MBA. Taking a leave of absence from medical school, Will opened his first biotech lab and serves as the chief science officer, writer, and innovator.

Will has founded and launched multiple biotech ventures while serving in a range of positions as chief executive officer, chief science officer, chief medical officer, founder, and innovator. His research-based protocols paved the way for wide-scale procedure use application in the medical field.

Many physicians and medical providers still use Will's protocols in their practice today, and have shared their success and techniques with hundreds of physicians and medical service providers.

For more information and to follow Will Bozeman's work, check out Longevity is the New Wellness Podcast on Apple Podcasts:

Longevity is the New Wellness | Podcasts on Audible | Audible.com

Made in the USA
Monee, IL
05 November 2026

67378695R00045